YOU AND YOUR V...

DR PATRICIA GILBER...
Medical Officer and a Medi...
munity Child Health. She w...
Hospital Medical School, London, and has both hospital
and general practice experience. She is also the author
of *Common Childhood Illnesses* (Sheldon Press), *Your
Pregnancy Diary* (Futura), *What Everywoman Should
Know About Her Breasts* (Sheldon Press) and co-author
of *The Complete Book of Babycare* (Octopus, Marks
and Spencer) and is a regular contributor to *Nursery
World*. She is married, with two children.

Overcoming Common Problems Series

The ABC of Eating
Coping with anorexia, bulimia and compulsive eating
JOY MELVILLE

Acne
How it's caused and how to cure it
PAUL VAN RIEL

An A–Z of Alternative Medicine
BRENT Q. HAFEN AND KATHRYN J. FRANDSEN

Arthritis
Is your suffering really necessary?
DR WILLIAM FOX

Birth Over Thirty
SHEILA KITZINGER

Body Language
How to read others' thoughts by their gestures
ALLAN PEASE

Calm Down
How to cope with frustration and anger
DR PAUL HAUCK

Common Childhood Illnesses
DR PATRICIA GILBERT

Coping with Depression and Elation
DR PATRICK McKEON

Curing Arthritis Cookbook
MARGARET HILLS

Curing Arthritis – The Drug-free Way
MARGARET HILLS

Depression
DR PAUL HAUCK

Divorce and Separation
ANGELA WILLANS

Enjoying Motherhood
DR BRUCE PITT

The Epilepsy Handbook
SHELAGH McGOVERN

Everything You Need to Know about Contact Lenses
DR ROBERT YOUNGSON

Everything You Need to Know about Your Eyes
DR ROBERT YOUNGSON

Everything You Need to Know about Shingles
DR ROBERT YOUNGSON

Family First Aid and Emergency Handbook
DR ANDREW STANWAY

Fears and Phobias
What they are and how to overcome them
DR TONY WHITEHEAD

Feverfew
A traditional herbal remedy for migraine and arthritis
DR STEWART JOHNSON

Fight Your Phobia and Win
DAVID LEWIS

Fit Kit
DAVID LEWIS

Flying Without Fear
TESSA DUCKWORTH AND DAVID MILLER

Goodbye Backache
DR DAVID IMRIE WITH COLLEEN DIMSON

Guilt
Why it happens and how to overcome it
DR VERNON COLEMAN

How to Bring Up your Child Successfully
DR PAUL HAUCK

How to Control your Drinking
DRS W. MILLER AND R. MUNOZ

How to Cope with Stress
DR PETER TYRER

Overcoming Common Problems Series

Overcoming Common Problems Series

Overcoming Common Problems

YOU AND YOUR VARICOSE VEINS

Dr Patricia Gilbert

M.B.B.S., M.R.C.S., L.R.C.P., D.R.C.O.G.

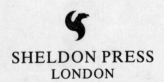

SHELDON PRESS
LONDON

First published in Great Britain in 1987 by
Sheldon Press, SPCK, Marylebone Road, London NW1 4DU

British Library Cataloguing in Publication Data

Gilbert, Patricia
  You and your varicose veins.—(Overcoming
common problems)
  1. Varicose veins
  I. Title   II. Series
  616.1′43   RC695

ISBN 0–85969–535–2
ISBN 0–85969–536–0 Pbk

Typeset by Deltatype, Ellesmere Port
Printed in Great Britain by
Richard Clay (The Chaucer Press) Ltd
Bungay, Suffolk

Contents

Introduction

Varicose veins are unknown in four-legged animals. So it is a fair assumption that one of the most important contributing factors in the cause of this common condition is our upright two-legged posture. There are, of course, many other factors involved, as not *every* upright human being suffers from varicose veins. Sex, race and inheritance all certainly play a part. And other factors such as weight, diet, exercise (or lack of it!) and pregnancy can all contribute to the presence, and severity, of varicose veins.

This book aims to give sufferers an insight into the causes of their problems based on simple anatomical and physiological explanations. The effects of varicose veins by way of aching legs, pain and pigmented skin as well as cosmetic appearance are discussed together with further, more serious, problems that can occur as complications of varicose veins.

Whilst varicose veins cannot be completely 'cured', there is much that can be done to alleviate the discomfort and improve the cosmetic appearance. Similarly, the onset of varicose veins cannot be prevented entirely. But with a few simple, sensible precautions and perhaps a change in life-style, the possibility of progression to more troublesome conditions can be avoided. For example, how about walking to the next bus-stop or tube station on the journey to work? Or how about joining a keep-fit session once a week instead of flopping in front of yet another television soap-opera every night? Both those activities will give your leg muscles some – probably much needed – work, and so help to pump the blood more efficiently through the circulatory system. You may also lose a kilo or two as a by-product of

1

the extra exercise. This, too, will ease the pressure on the veins of the legs as well as adding other health benefits.

Special conditions, such as pregnancy and long hours spent standing at work, for example, are also discussed in relationship to varicose veins. Other ways of reducing to a minimum the chances of these unsightly veins appearing will also be suggested.

I hope that this book will clear some of the misconceptions that have arisen in people's minds about varicose veins, both from the prevention and treatment angle. So put your best foot forward and show a shapely pair of lower limbs to the world throughout life!

1

How Varicose Veins Develop

Before looking at what goes wrong with veins to make them become varicose, we must look at the structure and function of normal veins. We must also view these important vessels in the context of the whole circulatory system – what they actually do, their relationship to arteries, capillaries and the heart itself.

The circulatory system

All organs and structures of the human body can be conveniently divided into 'systems'. Each of these systems fulfils a specific function. Examples of this division of labour, as it were, are in the renal system (consisting of kidney, ureters and bladder) which does the bulk of the work of eliminating waste products from our bodies. The digestive system (consisting of oesophagus, stomach, intestines and associated organs, such as the liver and the pancreas), responsible for taking in food and altering it to a convenient usable form, is another example of a bodily system. But it must be rememberd that every system is dependent on other organic systems and that no one part of the body works in isolation. The circulatory system is no exception.

The *function* of the circulatory system is to carry blood to and from all the tissues of the body. In this blood are carried oxygen and a wide variety of nutrients vital to the working of every other part of the body. In addition to this, waste products of metabolism are carried, in both gaseous and liquid form, to the organs of excretion. For example, in the blood there are waste substances carried to the kidneys. In the kidneys these waste products are processed to form

3

urine, which is then excreted outside the body. Similarly, the gaseous waste product of metabolism, carbon dioxide, is carried to the lungs where this unwanted gas is breathed out.

To fulfil these vital functions, the circulatory system consists of a network of arteries, capillaries and veins which permeate, in ever decreasing size, every tiniest cell of the body. Driving the blood continually round this network is the heart. Throughout life this incredible organ pumps, at an average of 70 beats per minute, blood around the miles (about 60,000!) of blood vessels.

The heart

This vital pump is an organ about the size of a grapefruit, situated in the chest. It is protected and surrounded on all sides by bone – the vertebral column at the back, the breastbone (or sternum) at the front and, completing the circle, the twelve pairs of ribs. The heart is made up of specialized muscle, known as cardiac muscle, which enables the pumping action to be kept going continuously throughout a lifetime.

For convenience of description, the heart can be thought of as a double pump working as a whole, but separated into two functional halves by a septum (partition) down the middle. Each half consists of two chambers. The *upper chamber* in each side is known as an atrium, or auricle, and is a collecting chamber. The right atrium receives back from the whole body blood which has lost its oxygen to the tissues (de-oxygenated blood). The left atrium receives blood back from the lungs where it has been re-oxgyenated by the process of respiration, or breathing in and out. The atria have, comparative to the lower chambers (or ventricles), thin walls. The ventricles (the lower chambers) are thick-walled and muscular. On them depend the pumping action which sends blood speeding round the body. The left ventricle, which receives back oxygenated blood from the lungs, pumps this blood around the body, whilst the right

HOW VARICOSE VEINS DEVELOP

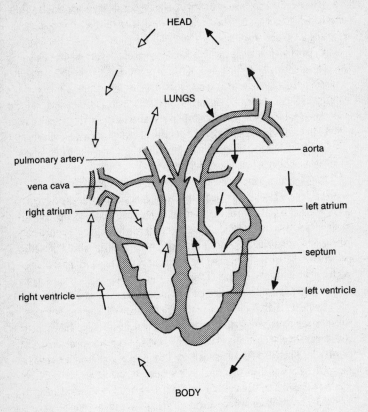

(arrows indicate direction of blood flow)

→ oxygenated blood
⇨ de-oxygenated blood

Fig. 1 Diagrammatic representation of heart

ventricle pushes the returned de-oxygenated blood through the lungs to pick up vital oxygen ready for re-cycling again to the tissues (see Figure 1 on p. 5.)

To perform its work the heart muscle itself requires an adequate supply of oxygen. This is provided by the coronary arteries, those tiny blood vessels no thicker than a piece of string. If these vital blood vessels become diseased and ultimately blocked (or thrombosed) the heart will be unable to continue its work. This is the situation that arises when a coronary thrombosis occurs – but that is another story only remotely connected to varicose veins!

This beautifully adapted pumping mechanism is controlled as to rate and force by intricate specialized nervous systems. Thus the rate and value can be adjusted to provide more blood – and hence oxygen and a higher rate of removal of waste products – when the body needs this as, for example, during exercise. Conversely, rate and force are reduced during rest and sleep.

To complete the picture of the heart, a brief word must be mentioned of the blood pressure, that important measurement that tells your doctor a good deal about the health of the circulatory system and other organs associated with its control. The blood pressure is the force exerted by each heart beat through the main arteries. It is measured as the force required to raise a column of mercury in the instrument known as a sphygnomanometer. The vast majority of people are familiar with this measuring device consisting of a wrap-around arm-band, attached to a device which reads the height of the column of mercury as the doctor or nurse listens with a stethoscope over a superficial artery. In a healthy young adult the heart beat raises the mercury level to 120mm. The lower figure of the blood pressure reading represents the resting pressure in the arteries and is also an important indication of the healthy function of the circulatory system.

So much for the heart, but what about those miles of blood vessels stretching into every corner of our bodies? How is their structure adapted to meeting differing needs?

The arteries

These are the blood vessels that carry the oxygenated blood from the left side of the heart to the rest of the body. One large vessel – the aorta – arises from the left ventricle. As it passes down through the body, smaller arteries are fed off to serve specific organs and structures, the aorta becoming smaller in size as this occurs. In the lower back region the aorta divides into two – into the iliac and then the femoral arteries – which pass down to feed the muscles, ligaments and bones of the legs. The walls of the arteries are thick, muscular and elastic to withstand the relatively high pressure inside their walls occurring at each beat of the heart. In good health, the inner walls of every artery are smooth. This allows blood to flow evenly through the vessel. (In later life, this smooth inner surface can become roughened, due to fatty deposits. This is one of the factors that predisposes blood to clot and so block, to a greater or lesser degree, the interior of a blood vessel.)

The arteries become progressively smaller and smaller as they extend further and further away from the heart until they are so minute that only a few blood corpuscles can pass through at any one time. At this stage they become known as *capillaries*. It is at the capillary level that the exchange of oxygen and nutrients to the tissues takes place. As the necessary oxygen and food are passed to the tissues, carbon dioxide and other waste products of metabolism are passed back from the tissues into the blood to be carried to the organs of excretion. The capillaries then join up again into tiny veins known as venules, which in turn gradually join to become the bigger veins.

The veins

These are the blood vessels that carry – in direct contrast to the arteries – de-oxygenated blood back to the heart ready for passage through the lungs to pick up oxygen again. The walls of veins are thinner and less elastic and muscular than those of the arteries. The pressure in these vessels is very much less than that in the arteries, and so – as ever in the structure of the human body – these vessels are perfectly adapted to their function. Again, the inner lining of the veins in health is smooth and allows the blood to pass along continuously and evenly.

Veins differ from arteries in one further way. At intervals along their length (and this is particularly important in the long veins of the leg as we shall see later) there are tiny one-way 'valves'. These 'valves' are rather like wings which, when closed, meet and fold together. Blood, once past these valves, cannot return into that portion of the vein through which it has already flowed. These valves and their correct functioning are the basis of the problems that can arise and lead to the presence of varicose veins, as will be seen later.

It is these vessels and their structure in the leg with which we are concerned as we look into the problem of varicose veins. Considering the length of the veins in the human leg it is perhaps surprising that problems with varicose veins do not arise more frequently. It can seem, at first sight, a minor miracle that blood can pass up about two feet of vein against gravity! And especially when it must be remembered that while the blood pressure in the arteries is equivalent to a force required to raise 120mm. mercury up a tube, this pressure has fallen dramatically to around 5mm. mercury by the time the blood reaches the capillary bed. So just how does the blood in your feet manage to return to your heart, and not just stagnate around your lower extremities – and particularly so when you are standing still?

There are four mechanisms by which the body ensures that the circulatory system is kept on the move from the feet up to the heart – in the upright adult, around a staggering four feet or so.

1　By far the most important is the massaging action of the muscles of the leg. Even when we are standing still the muscles of our legs are in a state of 'tone' – otherwise we would crumple up at the least breath of wind! And as we move, as in walking or running – and even changing from one foot to the other – the contraction, or tightening up of the muscles of the legs becomes firmer. This action squeezes the blood in the veins up towards the heart. But this is not the complete story of the beautifully adapted mechanism. The structure of the main muscles and tissues of the leg is such that a tough sheath of fibrous tissue encloses the bulk of the muscles. This sheath keeps the muscles tightly in control, and so increases the pressure of the contracting muscles on the veins situated deeply between them. (See later in this chapter on the relationship of deep and superficial veins to the bulky muscles of the leg.)

2　The positioning of the valves in the veins of the leg ensures that, even if the muscles slacken their pressure on the veins, the blood does not pass down the vein again. Once past a perfectly functioning valve there is no other way than onwards to the heart for the blood.

3　The very fact that, of necessity, the circulatory system is a closed circuit ensures that the blood is kept flowing in the correct direction. The pressure in the veins may be low, but nevertheless it is still a positive pressure urging the blood back to the heart. Obviously this pressure will assume more importance when we are lying down than when in the upright position. Standing up means that gravity will be acting against the return of the blood to the heart. But then, as we have seen, the muscles of the legs will counteract this effect.

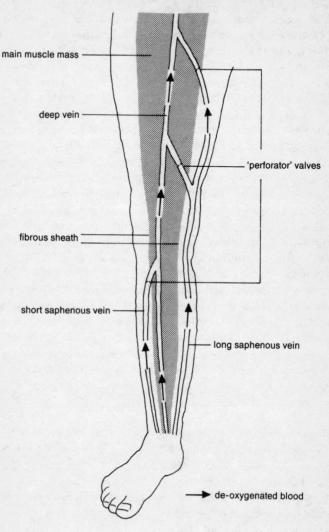

Fig. 2 Diagrammatic representation of venous drainage of leg

4 Remote as it may seem at first sight, our regular breathing mechanism also has an effect on the return of the blood to the heart. At each deep breath, a negative pressure occurs in the chest. And this has the beneficial effect of sucking the blood in the veins back up to the heart.

There is yet one more important aspect of anatomy that must be considered before we finally get to the subject of this book – varicose veins! And that is the relationship of the deep and superficial veins of the leg to the muscles and their tough, fibrous sheath.

The main vein draining the blood back from the muscles of the leg and foot into – finally – the heart is called the femoral vein. This vein is large in the region of the groin, but as it branches many times to gather blood from the large muscles of thigh and calf it becomes smaller – as with all vessels in the body as they approach the extremities. This system of veins is held in position deep in amongst the muscles, as we have seen, by a tough, fibrous sheath. The squeezing effect of the muscles therefore works very well in pushing the blood back up to the heart against gravity when we are in the upright position. (Obviously the flow is easily maintained when we are lying down, as the effect of gravity is non-existent from this viewpoint.) So – this system can be seen to be – almost – foolproof!

But what of the tissues – mainly fat and skin – outside the firm enclosing sheath of fibrous tissue? They, too, will need oxygen and nutrients carried to them in arteries and to have their waste products drained away by veins. To service these tissues there is the superficial or surface, system of veins. These veins have rather more muscular tissue in their walls than do the walls of the deep veins. With the help of this muscular tissue, these superficial veins can increase or decrease their size to accommodate changes in temperature or in response to injuries or to certain chemicals. Female sex hormones have a specific effect on the muscular walls of the veins. This is one factor why women tend to suffer more from varicose veins than do men (see Chapter 2).

Two main veins, again with many smaller sub-branches all the way up the leg, do this vital task. Up the inside of the leg runs the 'long saphenous' vein (saphenous meaning 'readily seen'), while the outside part of the calf is drained by the 'short saphenous' vein. These two veins perforate the fibrous sheath surrounding the muscles draining eventually into the main femoral vein. There are two main places where this perforation occurs. The long saphenous vein passes through the sheath in the region of the groin, whilst the short saphenous vein pierces the fibrous tissue behind the knee. There are also a number of smaller perforating veins along the length of the leg. Each 'perforation' has a valve at the point where it passes through the fibrous sheath. This valve – as with the other valves in the venous system – performs the important function of ensuring that the blood continues on its proper way – upwards – to the heart.

It is when these valves fail (due to a wide variety of possible causes – see Chapter 2) that varicose veins result. Blood from the deep veins of the leg gets pushed back – under pressure – into the smaller superficial veins of the saphenous system. The walls of these veins are unable to cope with this extra inrush of blood and over the years become dilated. Valves further back along this superficial system then fail, and then eventually – over many years – the bunches of swollen current-like veins become visible in the leg.

Recently some doubt has been cast as to whether or not it is an actual failure of the valves that is at the seat of the problem. It is postulated that it is the dilation of the veins themselves that is at fault. With a much distended vein it can be seen that the valves are just not large enough to block off the vessel and so prevent the blood from flowing backwards.

We shall see later (Chapter 2) that specific factors – female sex hormones, overweight and pregnancy, for example – cause an actual or relative dilation of the veins. So this theory of the actual mechanics of what causes varicose veins is certainly possible. Possibly some inherent differences in the make-up of the blood vessel walls in certain people could also have a bearing. This would fit in nicely with the familial tendency to varicose veins which is certainly a factor as to who will suffer from these problems. This is one more example of the fascinating detective work that occupies researchers in aspects of human disease.

From the description of the development of varicose veins, you can see that this is not an overnight occurrence. So you have no cause to worry that you will wake up one morning with a mass of varicose veins in your leg. And as will be seen later, many more years will elapse before any of the possible complications associated with varicose veins will occur. Also, with a few sensible precautions and possible early treatment, complications will never arise. The human leg veins need a little care (along with other parts of the body) as middle age approaches if they are efficiently to fulfil their function throughout a further thirty or forty years of life. Varicose veins cannot be entirely prevented. In the next chapter will be seen the possible reasons why they occur. Many of these pre-disposing conditions are quite outside our control. But with a little care and forethought, the worst effects of extensive varicose veins can be reduced to a minimum.

2

The Causes of Varicose Veins

We have seen, in the previous chapter, how varicose veins develop but are there any clues as to why this should happen in some people and not in others? A few facts about the incidence of varicose veins will help put the picture in perspective.

1 Sex

There is no doubt about it – women do suffer more from varicose veins than do men. Certainly women have a higher level of concern about the appearance of their legs than do men – after all who would *choose* to have the blue bumpy marks of varicose veins on their legs! And so, perhaps, women are more likely to seek treatment for their varicose veins than men. There is no doubt that this is partly the reason why hospital varicose veins clinics have a higher proportion of women than men. But this is not the whole reason. The condition really is more common in women. There are two probable reasons why this should be so:

The effect of female sex hormones

Oestrogen and progesterone are the hormones secreted by the ovaries that exert a great influence on the femininity of all women. These sex hormones also exert a specific effect on the veins of the body, the muscular walls being relaxed by their action. So the veins – and particularly those superficial veins on the legs which, as we have seen, have relatively more muscular tissue in their walls – become dilated with any rise in the level of the sex hormones. (Some women with varicose veins notice that their veins become painful at a

14

definite time during their menstrual cycle. This relates directly to the time in the normal cycle when the level of hormones is known to be high.)

The effect of pregnancy

Similarly, a further time in your life when varicose veins are likely to appear, or to worsen if you have them already, is during pregnancy. In part this is due to sex hormones again. Levels are high during pregnancy and so veins dilate, pressure increases and valves are more liable to fail. The problem in pregnancy is also compounded by the effect of the increased back pressure on the veins of your legs by your enlarging uterus. The larger the baby becomes the greater is the pressure on all the organs in the abdominal cavity. And this includes, of course, the veins draining the blood back to the heart from your legs. So, once again, the superficial veins have extra problems with which to cope – increased pressure from above as well as a general weakening of their walls. Fortunately, following the birth of your baby, the bulging, dilated veins will improve markedly with the lowering of the level of hormones and relief of the back pressure.

During pregnancy, too, varicose veins can develop around your vulval area (the area of the body surrounding the opening of the vagina) due to similar reasons which cause the development of varicose veins in your legs. Varicose veins in this situation will disappear soon after the birth of your baby.

It does seem slightly unfair that the sex who least enjoys the prospect of varicose veins should have, by very reason of her femininity, *two potent reasons* causing varicose veins.

Here is the case history of someone who had varicose veins in pregnancy.

*   *   *

It was Miranda's first baby. She and her husband Frank

15

were delighted to be becoming parents. Miranda had kept her antenatal appointments meticulously, had eaten a sensible diet and had kept up her twice weekly swimming sessions at the local baths. The pregnancy had gone smoothly, apart from an unpleasant few weeks of sickness during the first three months.

The only problem that was causing Miranda concern when the time came for her to leave her job as a secretary in one of the local building societies was the varicose veins that had gradually appeared in the calf of her left leg. As her baby grew in size, so did her varicose veins – or so it seemed to Miranda.

As she stood doing the ironing one morning, the dull ache in her left leg really began to get her down. And when her mother arrived for a mid-morning cup of coffee, Miranda burst into tears.

'Whatever is the matter, Miranda? – aren't you feeling well? Come and sit down, love,' Mrs Butler took her daughter's arm and led her to the settee. 'Sit down and put your feet up.'

'Look at these awful varicose veins, Mum,' sobbed Miranda. 'They look so ugly – and – and – they *do* ache. I don't suppose they will ever go away now.'

'Is *that* what is worrying you?' Mrs Butler's face showed her relief. 'All the family have had varicose veins when they were pregnant – and look – mine are hardly noticeable now, and that is after four children! You show Dr Pearce at your next antenatal visit – he will give you some advice.'

The following day Miranda asked to see her doctor. She showed him her leg, and confessed that she had been upset about the bulging blue veins that marred the smooth contour of her calf.

'Three things to do, Miranda,' Dr Pearce said briskly. 'Put your feet up as much as possible whenever you are sitting down. Walk to the shops or to the park every day. Wear the support stocking I am going to prescribe for you.' As he started to write the prescription pad, Dr Pearce looked at Miranda and smiled; 'No, not three things to do – four. And the fourth one is – don't worry! When your baby is born, those veins will be much improved – in fact you'll hardly notice them.'

Miranda's baby boy, William, was born six weeks later. Within a few days Miranda was home revelling in her new motherhood role. At her post-natal examination when William was six weeks old, Dr Pearce said: 'Let me have a look at your legs and see how those varicose veins are that caused you so much distress.'

'Oh – I had quite forgotten about them.' And Miranda looked down at the calf of her left leg. 'Goodness – you can hardly see where they were! Just a faint mark – there and there.' Miranda traced with her finger the faint blue line down the inside of her leg.

'You didn't believe me did you when I said they would improve after your baby was born. But keep up the walking – and start wearing your support stocking early on in your next pregnancy!' Dr Pearce smiled at Miranda as she bent to pick up William in his Moses basket. 'He's worth a varicose vein or two, isn't he?'

Miranda did not need to reply. The shine in her eyes as she looked down at her little son was sufficient answer.

*   *   *

2 Family history

If you want to avoid varicose veins, choose your family carefully! It is a fact that if your mother, grandmother, aunts or cousins suffer from varicose veins, you are also more likely to follow in the family pattern than if no one in the family carried these blemishes on their legs.

Varicose veins are certainly not inherited in the same way as, for example, are blue or brown eyes or certain abnormalities or diseases, such as colour-blindness or haemophilia. But, just as our bodily configuration and personality traits all show a familial pattern, so does the tendency to varicose veins. The actual structure of the blood vessels, and possibly the structure of the valves in the veins also, is important from a familial view-point.

Nothing can be done about these basic anatomical and physiological tendencies. But if you are aware of the possibility of certain conditions, such as varicose veins occurring, you can take certain steps to at least reduce the severity of the symptoms.

This leads directly on to the third possible causative factor – or factors – in the incidence of varicose veins – namely, our Western life-style.

3 Life-style

Under this heading comes the oft-discussed questions of overweight, exercise and diet. While all these three factors are very much interwoven, let us look at them each in turn:

Overweight

While being overweight will not cause varicose veins, the excess load on the veins of the legs will certainly cause any existing varicose veins to become more dilated and tortuous. Treatment of varicose veins, too, in overweight people is always a potential nightmare. For example, firm bandaging of the legs following injection or surgical treatment is more difficult. In addition, the doctor has to wade through mounds of fat on the legs to find the source of the problem. Add to this the fact that most overweight people are less likely to take adequate exercise, as well as eating too much for their needs, and you can see that overweight is a definite factor in the severity of varicose veins. (See Chapter 6 on ideal weight ranges and suggestions on how to reach – and stick at! – your ideal weight.)

Exercise

A high proportion of workers in the Western world have sedentary jobs. Sitting at a desk all day, having been transported to work in a sitting position and going home to sit for several hours in front of the television, does nothing at all to make the muscles of the leg work. And we have seen, in a previous chapter, the importance of the massaging action of the muscles of the leg in propelling the blood in the veins up to the heart. Ideally we should all walk at least two or three miles a day – not just a saunter around the shops, but a brisk 'stepping-out' walk. In a later chapter, it will be seen that this very thing is of vital importance in the successful treatment of varicose veins.

Diet

As well as playing a prime part in the control of overweight, our type of diet also plays a large part in our bowel function, which in turn can have an effect on the incidence of varicose veins. Western diets have an emphasis on refined foods with only a minimal amount of roughage, or fibre. The result of this in many people is a chronic state of constipation. (It is well known that constipation over many years can lead to diverticular disease in the lower bowel. This condition means that there are small balloon-like 'blow-outs' in the large bowel which can on occasions become infected and cause pain and diarrhoea. But that, again, is another story . . .) Hard masses of waste material are retained for comparatively long periods in the lower bowel. It is possible that these masses exert sufficient pressure on the large veins in the pelvis to cause back pressure on the veins of the leg. And this in turn can cause dilation of veins and possible damage to valves in the lower leg. Constipated people, too, often pass their motions with much straining. This also increases the pressure on veins with, again, potential damaging results to weak or already damaged blood vessels.

It is a well-documented fact that African people who eat a diet rich in fibre, rarely suffer from constipation. They also have a far lower incidence of varicose veins although they are not completely unknown. Other factors of life-style, such as more exercise and little chance of being overweight, obviously also have a bearing on the relative immunity to varicose veins of these peoples.

So, no one factor in this trilogy accounts entirely for the onset of varicose veins. They are all very much interrelated. (And varicose veins are only one problem which possibly results from our Western life-style. Perhaps we should all look into the diet, exercise and weight aspects of our daily lives, not only to avoid the discomfort of varicose veins, but many other conditions as well.)

There are two further factors which people often think are of possible importance in the onset of varicose veins, but which, in reality, have little effect on the appearance of these blemishes.

Long hours of standing

Many occupations require people to stand all day. Hairdressing, some forms of factory work, serving in shops, are but a few examples of this. In itself, these activities will not produce varicose veins *if* the superficial veins of the leg are healthy with competent valves. But if one or several of the factors previously discussed apply, the chances of varicose veins developing are higher. And, of course, if you are already a sufferer from varicose veins, your occupation will probably increase the severity of your varicose veins. If this is the problem in your particular situation, try gently rocking back and forwards on your feet at regular intervals during the day, walking a few yards whenever possible or just contracting the muscles of your calves now and again. This will help, to some extent, in improving the blood flow in the veins of your legs. (The latter trick is also one employed by guardsmen or soldiers on duty to counteract any tendency to fainting in, for example, very hot weather. The tightening up of the muscles of the leg – without actually moving – has the effect of ensuring adequate return of blood to the heart for further circulation.)

Tight garters or 'hold-up' stockings

The effect of any constriction around the leg will increase the pressure in the veins below the constriction. Once again, this marginal increase in back pressure is one which healthy superficial leg veins will probably be able to cope with. So again, varicose veins will not actually be *caused* by the wearing of this constrictive type of clothing. But if varicose veins are already a problem, it is sensible to avoid such constrictions.

So, an ideal situation in which to find yourself (if you were to have the choice) avoiding varicose veins is:

1 to be born a male;
2 into a family in whom varicose veins were unknown;
3 to lead an active, non-sedentary life;
4 eating a diet high in roughage and low in refined foods.

There is little we can do about the first two factors. But there are measures which can mitigate the last two factors (see Chapter 6).

3

How Varicose Veins Affect
Your Life

Having seen how varicose veins develop and considered some of the factors that are thought to be involved in their appearance, just how will they affect your life? There can be other problems in your legs that can cause trouble, and occasionally these symptoms can be confused with those due to varicose veins. But first of all a run-down on those signs and symptoms all too familiar to you if you have varicose veins.

1   The *appearance* of your legs. Varicose veins on the calves and behind the knees (the most common place for them to appear) certainly do *not* enhance the visual impact of a shapely pair of legs! But, as with many other – often relatively minor – blemishes on the body, varicose veins are often far less noticeable to other people than you think. So, while it is always a good policy to obtain your doctor's advice about any deviation from the normal – for you – in any part of your body, do not be surprised at his negative response if you attend with one small varicose vein. Masterly inactivity is probably the most common 'treatment' for early minor degrees of varicose veins.

2   *Aching legs* can sometimes result from varicose veins, and particularly so if you are on your feet all day long. The lack of drainage of blood back to your heart from your legs can make them feel tired, heavy and achy. There are many other causes of aches and pains in your legs, and so it is a good idea to ask your doctor's advice if you have aching legs. He, or she, will be able – by asking you questions about the type of pain and its timing as well as examining your legs – to

sort out the ache due to varicose veins from other problems that can cause pain or discomfort in the legs. (See later in this chapter for other causes of pain in the legs.)

3   Then, finally, other signs and symptoms of varicose veins which will send you post-haste to your doctor will be one or the other of the *complications* that can result. There are four main complications that *can* occur due to the presence of varicose veins:

- haemorrhage (following on from injury)
- phlebitis
- pigmentation
- ulceration

These complications, it must be stressed, are by *no means* an inevitable outcome of varicose veins. Also do remember that these more serious aspects of varicose veins only occur after many years (see Chapter 5). So there are comparatively few signs and symptoms associated with varicose veins. But, nevertheless, varicose veins can have an impact on your life-style in many ways.

Your job

If you have ambitions to be a model or to win beauty contests, it might be as well to reconsider your options if you suffer from varicose veins! Any hint of dilated bluish markings on the smooth contour of calves and thighs and any employer or judge will politely pass on to the next candidate or entrant.

Work, too, which entails long hours of standing should, if at all possible, be avoided if varicose veins are present in any degree of severity. Such occupations do not *cause* varicose veins, but if minor degrees of varicose veins are present, standing still for hours on end will certainly not improve them. Occupations which include a good deal of walking around do not, of course, fall into this category. The massaging effect of the active muscles of the leg during walking gives valuable assistance to adequate return of blood to the heart. It is the long hours of standing in one position – at a factory bench or behind a shop-counter with little chance of movement – that can cause varicose veins to become more pronounced, and also more uncomfortable.

Your contraceptive

Much has been written, over the years, about the oral method of contraception. 'The pill' is probably the most well-known tablet ever to be swallowed by women. Much research has gone into the effectivity of different types of oral contraceptives, and also into any possible adverse side-effects resulting from years of using this form of contraception. When one considers that there are probably around 3 million women in Britain taking oral contraceptives for many years of their lives, it is no wonder that the pill is a much-researched product.

There are several types of oral contraceptive pills. The majority are made up of a mixture of two hormones found naturally in the female body – oestrogen and progesterone. Different oral contraceptives have varying amounts of these two hormones amd most women will find out by trial and error which one suits them best. They act by preventing the release of the ovum (or egg) from the ovary each month.

Initially – about forty years ago – the oral contraceptive pills consisted mainly of the hormone oestrogen. And very effective it was at preventing the release of eggs from the ovary. But after a couple of decades of use, it came to the notice of the medical profession that some young women were suffering from clotting in their arteries and veins. Heart attack, strokes and thrombosis in the deep veins of the leg were being reported in an age group in which such events

24

were previously rare. The numbers were not high, but of sufficient size to warrant further enquiry into the possible cause. Further research led to the belief that the oestrogen in the contraceptive pill could be a factor. So the oestrogen component in the pill was reduced and the progesterone proportion increased. This was found to be equally effective from a contraception viewpoint, but with less risk of producing clotting in the blood vessels. The risks of 'clotting' due to modern oral contraceptives are infinitesimal – far, far less than the risk you take every time you cross the road!

But what has all this to do with varicose veins? Again, the difference must be stressed between women who already have varicose veins, and the woman who has none of these blemishes on her legs. There is no evidence at all to show that there is any connection between taking the oral contraceptive pill and the appearance of varicose veins if you previously had none. But if you already suffer from varicose veins your doctor will think it inadvisable to start you on the oral contraceptive pill. Once existing varicose veins have been adequately treated, however, the pill can again be prescribed, after a wait of a month or two.

Similarly, if you have any history of either clotting in a deep vein or phlebitis (an inflammation around a vein), the oral contraceptive pill is not for you – because of the danger (albeit small) of further clotting episodes.

Again, doctors are reluctant to prescribe oral contraceptives to women over thirty-five years of age. Clotting over this age becomes relatively more common, and so any further risk is not justified. Smoking, of course, also adds further clotting hazards, so if you smoke and are over thirty-five years old, your doctor will certainly not want to prescribe the contraceptive pill for you.

The following case history highlights the problems of varicose veins and the pill.

*   *   *

'It's nice to have had your children young – but it doesn't do much for your ego when you attend the same family planning clinic as your married daughter!' Beth Williams settled back in the chair of her friend's house as they took time out from arranging the local NSPCC's fund-raising event.

'And especially when she was given the Pill without question,' Beth continued, 'and I was told it was inadvisable to continue with it at my age!'

Judy Fleetwood took a long drink of her welcome cup of tea. 'I know the feeling well, Beth,' she said, 'but my reasons for not having the Pill were different from yours.'

'All right – I know you are about fifteen years younger than me,' laughed Beth. 'What's your problem, then?' she added.

'My varicose veins,' said Judy, flatly. 'My mother had them, my grandmother had them and even old Uncle Jim had a sizeable crop. So I really did not stand much chance of avoiding them.'

'So what has that got to do with the contraceptive pill?' asked Beth in a puzzled voice.

'Well – apparently it could be dangerous to take the Pill if you have severe varicose veins – which mine certainly are.' Judy pointed to several blue swellings over the inside of the calf of the left leg. 'They appeared first when I was working in that dress shop, and got much worse when I was carrying the twins.'

'Does it mean, then, that you will never be able to take the Pill?' asked Beth.

'No, when my veins have been treated I can go on the Pill,' replied Judy, 'and I've been lucky. There has been a cancellation at St Luke's from next week, and so I've accepted the bed and will be having the operation on my veins Thursday of next week. Brian's Mum is coming to look after the twins.'

Three weeks later, Beth and Judy were finalizing the accounts of the NSPCC fête. Judy, sitting with her bandaged leg up on a chair, said: 'I'll be able to go on the Pill in three months' time, Beth. I went to the family planning clinic today.'

'Lucky old you!' replied Beth. 'There's no chance of having an operation to improve my age, I'm afraid,' she added, glumly. 'But you can't have everything – I'm fortunate not to have varicose veins.'

*   *   *

Maybe neither of these circumstances apply to you, but perhaps it is their nuisance value that leads you to seek advice. The complications that can arise in a few unfortunate sufferers are, of course, quite a different problem. But before looking at the treatment available for varicose veins, a brief look at other conditions that can give rise to pain and discomfort in your legs. Your doctor will want to eliminate these causes before sending you off to have your varicose veins treated. It is a waste of time and effort as well as disappointing for you, if your discomfort is not relieved after treatment – and all because the root of the trouble was not due to varicose veins after all.

Cramp

This is a painful tightening of the muscles, frequently those in the calf of the leg, with which many of us are familiar. This cramp comes on quite out of the blue and can be excruciating while it lasts. Many are the theories that have been put forward as to its cause. But few of these theories hold water when looked into in more depth. Fortunately these painful spasms last only a few minutes. Rubbing the affected part, or deliberately stretching the muscle that is in spasm does seem to hasten relief.

Leg cramps seem particularly prone to occur in older people and also during pregnancy. The spasms often seem to disappear quite spontaneously, to possibly recur again in a year or two for a while. There do not seem to be any long-lasting effects from even frequent attacks of leg cramp.

The pain is quite different from the aching, 'heavy' pain associated with varicose veins. But unless you are aware of its existence, you may possibly lay the blame at the door of your varicose veins.

'Intermittent claudication'

This is a very grand-sounding name for disease in the arteries of the leg. When these arteries become narrowed through disease, less blood is able to pass along these vessels. So the muscles are virtually being starved of oxygen and nutrients. This is fine when you are putting no muscular demands on your legs. But when your muscles have work to do, as in walking, climbing stairs or any other sustained activity, they protest – violently! A cramp-like pain will be felt in the affected muscles and you will be forced to stand still. After a few minutes the pain passes, as the muscles once again receive an adequate supply of oxygen. But if the 'work' is begun again the pain returns – due to the same cause – lack of an adequate blood supply to the tissues of the leg.

An accurate description of these symptoms will give your doctor the clue to the true diagnosis of what is causing the leg pain. This is, once more, a pain quite unlike that associated with varicose veins but, again, one that could be confused with it if you are unaware of the possibilities.

Arthritis

There are two main types of arthritis – quite different from each other. *Osteo-arthritis* is the condition – usually found in older people – in which the ends of the bones, inside the joint, become damaged. This is the result of the stresses and strains on these weight-bearing joints over many years of, perhaps strenuous, use. The cartilage covering the ends of the bones is destroyed. So the surfaces of the bones rub together. And this is painful! Knees and hips are the joints commonly affected. Unless careful examination of the joints is undertaken, the pain felt down in the lower part of the leg can be thought to be due to varicose veins.

Rheumatoid arthritis is the other arthritic condition which could be confused with pain due to varicose veins. But this is less likely – for several reasons. The cause of this form of arthritis is still not completely understood, and it is probable that a variety of factors is involved. But this disease affects younger people – women more than men – and affects more frequently the smaller joints of the body, such as fingers, wrists and ankles. In severe cases, the larger joints, such as knees, are also involved. So the pattern of the disease is such that the ache due to varicose veins is rarely confused.

But your doctor will soon be able correctly to diagnose the cause of the pain in your legs.

Slipped disc or sciatica

Between the bones of the vertebral column are slim wedges of cartilage. These can be pushed out of place by excess stresses and strains on the vertebral column – yet one more penalty of the upright posture. When this happens, the nerve next to the displaced cartilage is squeezed, and acute pain is transmitted down this nerve to the muscle. As the inter-vertebral discs most frequently affected are in the region of the lower back, the large nerve known as the sciatic nerve is frequently affected – hence the name 'sciatica'. The pain of sciatica passes down the back of the leg – as any sufferer will tell you – and on down into the calf. This pain is acute and quite unlike the dull ache of varicose vein discomfort. Again, your doctor will be able to tell from the description of your symptoms the most likely cause of your problem. A simple test – raising the affected leg up as you lie on your back – will further clarify the diagnosis. If you have a slipped disc, the pain will become acute as your leg is raised 30° or so from the horizontal. The discomfort due to varicose veins will not be affected at all by this test.

There are other, less common causes, for pain in the legs, but the four described are the conditions which could possibly make you think that it was your varicose veins that were giving problems.

Two other conditions deserve a brief mention.

'Fidgety' legs

Older women occasionally complain that they have restless legs – especially in the evenings, and when they are sitting quietly by the fireside. Pain is not a problem, but just the uncomfortable, irritating feeling in the legs that they must continually be moved in an attempt to get comfortable.

Poor drainage of blood in the lower legs is thought to be the cause of this irritating symptom. Your doctor will be able to prescibe medication if you find this symptom too uncomfortable. But try taking a short walk at intervals and then sitting with your legs raised to at least a position horizontal with your body and preferably higher than this. These simple measures may well improve your symptoms.

'Broken' veins or 'spider naevi'

These are the tiny, red, thread-like veins that appear on the thighs and calves of some women. (And occasionally on cheeks and nose.) They are nothing to do with varicose veins, but just tiny dilated veins which are particularly near the surface of the skin. They can often first make their appearance during pregnancy – and will often persist throughout life.

Little can be done to 'cure' these tiny blemishes. The best that you can do is to use one of the excellent cover-up creams available if they are causing you too much embarrassment.

These then are the signs and symptoms associated with varicose veins, and those conditions in the leg that could possibly be confused with them. The next chapter will describe the treatment that is available for varicose veins.

4

The Treatment of Varicose Veins

The *treatment* of simple varicose veins (i.e. those varicosities in which none of the complications have intervened) obviously depends on their severity. Your own general practitioner must be your first line of help if you are concerned about either the appearance of, or symptoms associated with, your varicose veins. Again, depending on the severity, he will decide whether or not to refer you to a surgeon for advice and possible treatment. (Because varicose veins are such a common problem, in many parts of the country there are often long waiting lists for both consultation and treatment. So often simple measures to relieve symptoms are tried first.)

There are four main ways of tackling the problem of varicose veins:

1 to do nothing;
2 to use, on a regular basis, support stockings;
3 injection treatment;
4 surgical treatment.

No treatment

This is not as negative as it sounds. Your doctor, with his extensive experience of the varying degrees of severity of varicose veins, will be able to reassure you that your particular veins are not in any immediate danger of progressing to complications. He will also be able to give you advice on what you can do to avoid, as far as possible, your varicosities from worsening. (See Chapter 6 on self-help measures.)

So do not be annoyed or irritated that there is a negative response from your doctor to what are, to you, those very ugly blemishes on your legs. With minor degrees of varicosities, treatment would not benefit you greatly. But do remember to seek your doctor's advice again if (in spite of all your self-help measures) your varicose veins do become markedly worse over the next few years. As we have seen, many of the factors involved in the incidence of varicose veins are quite beyond your control – after all, very few people indeed can change their sex, and no one can change their family! And it is these factors that play a significant part in the incidence of varicose veins. So it is possible that in a few years' time, treatment will be appropriate for you.

Support stockings

To be strictly accurate, support stockings cannot be classed as a 'treatment' for varicose veins. The word 'treatment' implies a procedure that results in a cure for the condition under treatment – in the case of varicose veins, either injection or surgical treatment.

Nevertheless, very many people wear support stockings because of their varicose veins. These aids are of value in a number of circumstances:

1 During *pregnancy*. Varicose veins, as has been seen, can either become apparent for the first time during pregnancy or become worse during the latter months. The main factor involved here is the back pressure on the veins of your legs by your developing baby. When this pressure is relieved following the birth of your baby, the varicose veins will show a marked improvement, although they will never disappear completely.

2 For use whilst *awaiting further treatment*. As long as there are waiting-lists for treatment (either injection or surgery)

for varicose veins there will be a need for support stockings. Definitely not a curative measure (see later for 'mode of action'), but much comfort can be obtained from wearing support stockings.

3 Following *injection or surgical treatment*. Support stockings are an important part of the after-care of the legs following definitive treatment (see later in this chapter).

4 Following *successful treatment of one of the complications of varicose veins*. Support stockings are of particular value in the after-care of people who have suffered from either a leg ulcer due to varicose veins or have had clotting and/or inflammation of one of the deep veins of the leg. After the initial complication has been treated, support stockings can do much – along with other measures – to reduce to a minimum the possibility of recurrence. Also much comfort – an important factor – will be felt by wearing this form of hosiery.

5 For *elderly*, or *people too unwell* for other forms of treatment. Even though treatment for varicose veins is a relatively minor procedure, it can be inadvisable to submit older people (who may have other more serious conditions as well) to a general anaesthetic which is usually necessary for surgical procedure. Also, as will be seen later, regular walking is a vital part of the after-care of either injection or surgical treatment. This may just not be possible for older people or those people who suffer from other conditions that make walking either impossible or difficult.

How support stockings work

What support stockings do is very simple. The firm control these aids exert on the tissues of the leg helps to squeeze blood into the deep veins of the leg. This in turn is passed back up the venous system into the heart. So the dilated, weakened varicose veins of the superficial system will gain prime benefit from this action. And especially so during walking, when the action of the muscles on the deep veins of the leg assists in the whole process of returning blood to the heart.

If your daily work requires you to stand for long hours, support stockings will do much to stop the blood stagnating in the dilated veins of the superficial system. But remember that to get the full advantage of support stockings the 'muscle-pump' of your calf muscles should be used. So even if you cannot walk far during your day's work, try at least to walk a few yards as often as you can.

When you sit down for a few minutes during the day's work, try and prop your legs up on a chair or stool. In this way the return of blood from your legs is not having to overcome gravity. So there is much less back pressure on the dilated veins, with their weakened walls, of your legs.

There is no need – and indeed no benefit – in wearing your support stockings at night or if you are resting in bed for any period of time. While you are in a horizontal position, gravity is not working against the upward movement of the blood in your veins. And even better than lying horizontal is to be lying with your legs above the level of your heart. Venous blood from your lower extremities can then flow with a fair degree of ease back to the heart. To achieve this either raise the end of your bed up – with wooden blocks for example – or put your feet and lower legs on a pillow or two. (Obviously, if you are elderly and/or have any heart condition which necessitates you resting in a sitting or half-sitting position, this procedure may well be impossible. Under these circumstances, check with your doctor, or district nurse, as to what is best for you.)

Remember to avoid any hard – or too firm – object pressing into any part of your leg. Any kinking of the superficial vein can cause back pressure on your varicose veins – which is the very situation you are trying to avoid. Similarly it is always best to avoid crossing your legs – either at knee or ankle level – when lying in bed. This again causes unnecessary back pressure on weakened veins. (And this also applies, of course, to crossing legs when sitting – such a common procedure. Notice how many of your friends and colleagues automatically cross their legs as they sit!)

Obtaining your support stockings

These can be bought over the counter in any chemist or surgical appliance shop without prescription. Alternatively your own doctor or hospital consultant can prescribe support stockings for you. This latter method of obtaining support stockings is necessary when you are outside the standard range – for example, if you are extra tall. Under these circumstances it is necessary to have accurate measurements in order that the support will be of value. This prescription can be taken to a surgical appliances shop or can be obtained from the appropriate department at your local hospital.

There are a few points about support stockings that must be remembered if they are to do an adequate job:

1   The *elasticity* of the support must be adequate. In other words the pressure exerted on the superficial leg veins must be of a certain level, otherwise very little benefit is obtained. Stockings come in a range of elasticity, those with the firmest control exerting a pressure equivalent to that required to raise 60mm. of mercury when correctly fitted and applied. Stockings exerting a pressure of less than that required to raise 30mm. of mercury are of little value. (Pressure in many aspects of medical measurement – for example, blood-pressure – is frequently measured in terms of millimetres of mercury. So do not get confused by thinking that mercury will be an integral part of your support stocking!)

A word of caution here about support tights that can be bought in many chemists. While these can be of comfort to tired aching legs, they will not give sufficient pressure necessary to aid the return of blood from dilated varicose veins. By all means wear them if you find them comfortable and of help in supporting the muscles of your leg (and this they do very well). But as a long-term treatment for varicose veins you should be looking for a firmer support.

2   Support stockings should be *open at the toe*. Toes can become extremely uncomfortable if squeezed together tightly by a firm elastic stocking. Remember, too, that there is much movement going on at the joints where your toes meet the main part of your foot. Everytime you take a step these joints bend almost at a right angle. And anything that restricts this movement will cause discomfort and possible damage to joints and blood vessels. Support stockings should start *above* the joints connecting the toes to the main part of the foot.

3   *Length* of support stocking. Support stockings come in two lengths – one full-length and one up to the knee. The type which is most suitable for you will be dependent upon where your varicose veins are situated. If you only have varicose veins on the lower part of your leg, your doctor or surgeon will probably consider that a below-knee support will be adequate for you. These are self-supporting and will tuck neatly into the part of your leg immediately above the bulge of the calf, and below the knee.

If, however, there are varicosities in the thighs, a full-length support is necessary. These will need some form of control to ensure they are kept in the correct position. Suspenders are suitable for women. Men will need to wear a waist-support of some kind to hold the stockings up – a suspender attached to a button on the inside of the waist-band of the trousers can also successfully perform this function.

4   The *material* from which the support stockings is made should, as well as having the right degree of elasticity, be sufficiently porous to allow perspiration to evaporate. Moist,

hot skin overlying an area of the leg which has poor venous drainage is an added, unnecessary, hazard in the possibility of the development of a varicose ulcer (see Chapter 5).

So now you have support stockings. How are you to use them to gain maximum effect?

1   *When* to wear support stockings. The benefits of support stockings occur when the blood in the veins of the leg is having to work against gravity in order to return to the heart – that is, when we are standing up. Therefore, support stockings should be worn throughout the day, and not at night when a horizontal position in bed is maintained.

It is most important, however, that support stockings are put on *before* your feet touch the floor in the mornings. Reach for your stockings before getting out of bed and pull them on carefully before you swing your legs off your mattress. By doing this there will be no blood trapped in the dilated veins of the superficial system. Maximum effect in keeping the blood moving in these veins will thus be obtained.

2   *How* to put on support stockings. A little talcum powder is of great help in performing this task. So remember to have this available ready at hand beside your support stocking so that you need not get out of bed until your stocking is fulfilling its function.

Smooth a little of the talc over the whole surface of your leg (or legs if both are involved). Roll the stocking from the top down until you can firmly hold the whole stocking in a stretched position over your toes. Ease this over your toes until the lower end of the stocking is at the level of the base of your toes. Gently pull the stocking up to its correct level, smoothing out any creases as you go. It is important that there are no kinks or bulges which can press into the veins and obstruct the upward flow of blood.

Finally, make sure that your stocking is firmly attached – if you are wearing a full length one – to a couple of suspenders. Also be sure that it feels comfortable, and that the pressure on your leg feels consistent – no tight ridges at the knee or toe for example.

An ordinary stocking or pair of tights can be pulled on over the support stocking for appearance sake. If you are wearing trousers, a pair of suitable socks to protect your feet will probably be all that you need.

3 *Care* of your support stockings. These should be washed as frequently as you wash other stockings or tights in warm, soapy water. They should be dried flat after removing excess water by rolling them in a dry towel. Never hang support stockings over a radiator to dry. This will ruin the elasticity and shape.

Check at regular intervals, every month or so, the elasticity of your stockings. With frequent – necessary – washings this elasticity will deteriorate. (You will probably also notice as the weeks pass that you are not getting so much support.) Most good quality stockings will last around six months or so. But do not forget to obtain a replacement well in advance of the stockings becoming floppy. Unless support stockings give adequate pressure, they are doing no good at all.

As well as being used as the sole treatment for varicose veins, support stockings play an important role in the after-care of varicose veins that have undergone either injection or surgical treatment. The basic facts of choice of stocking, method of using and care of stockings will also apply if the stockings are used as an adjunct to other forms of treatment.

Injection treatment

This is perhaps the treatment with which most people are familiar. One only has to look round at the legs in a crowded supermarket to see how many people – particularly women – are wearing bandages covered by support stockings. And many of these will be in this condition as part of the follow-up to injection treatment.

How injection treatment works

The basic idea behind this form of treatment is to block off completely the vein that has become varicosed – thus eliminating altogether the disfiguring swelling. This is done by injecting a very small amount of irritant fluid into the affected vein. A controlled inflammation is thus set up. The end result of this is the formation of scar tissue. This effectively blocks off the particular vein so that blood does not flow backwards into the damaged vein. (Adequate blood can still be returned from the area of the leg involved via other healthy veins.) Care must be taken when giving the injection that the right amount is injected into the correct position. This ensures that the intense inflammation set up will be controlled and limited only to the site of the varicosed vein.

There are a number of different fluids that can be injected and each surgeon will have his own particular favourite. But the basic principles are the same whatever product is used.

How this treatment will affect you

1 *At the time* depending on local circumstances, you will either be given injection treatment at your initial visit, once the doctor has decided that this is the appropriate treatment for your particular varicose veins. Or – and this is probably more usual – you will be given a further appointment to return to the hospital clinic when an injection session is in progress.

So now you have actually arrived in the clinic, and after probably many months of waiting and wondering, the time has arrived for you to see the last – hopefully – of your varicose veins.

THE TREATMENT OF VARICOSE VEINS

First of all, the doctor will need to determine exactly where he is going to give his injection. This must be given into the vein which perforates the fibrous sheath separating the deep venous system from the superficial venous system – the 'perforator vein'. But before this, he will need to mark out on the skin of your leg the full extent of the varicosities. This must be done in the standing position because, as varicose veins sufferers will be well aware, it is in the upright position these veins are at their most prominent.

Having done this, you will be asked to lie down and your leg will be raised so that the varicose veins are emptied by gravity. When this is done little indentations can be seen – and felt. These are the positions where the 'perforators' are situated – and hence the place (or places) where the doctor must inject the irritant fluid. To check that the right position, or positions, have been established, you will be asked to stand again, this time with the doctor's finger controlling the perforating vein. If the position is correct, there will be no bulging of the vein as the upright position is attained. A further mark will be made on your skin to pin-point the exact position of the injection.

You lie down on the couch again, and a specially firm compression bandage will be applied to your leg, starting at your toes and winding closely up to immediately below the site of the varicose vein which is under treatment. With your leg raised slightly above the horizontal, a small amount of the fluid is injected into the appropriate place. (The needle used is a very fine one, and you will feel the minimum of pain – hardly worse than the prick of a pin or needle on your finger – in fact less so, as this part of your leg is comparatively poorly supplied with pain-feeling nerves.) A dry sterile dressing is then placed over the site of the injection. The firm bandage will then be continued up to your knee. A support stocking is then pulled on over this bandage – and all this is finished!

But the success of the treatment will very much depend on:

a *Bandaging* The compression bandage that has been wound on to your leg at the time of the injection procedure *must* be kept in place for fully six weeks. If you are having difficulties with this, perhaps by way of slipping or becoming wrinkled, return either to your doctor or to the varicose vein clinic at the hospital. Here the nurse will be able to reapply the bandage for you.

Remember, too, that you must not get this bandage wet. So a long soak in the bath is not for you for a while! Either a good wash, or a shower with a large plastic bag tightly encasing your bandaged leg must be your way of keeping clean for a while. (Some agile people can manage to have a bath in a minimum of water by swinging their bandaged leg over the side of the bath. But most people have to think of other ways of keeping clean.)

b *Exercise* This is probably the single most important factor in the successful treatment of varicose veins. You should walk – briskly – for at least three miles *every* day. And this means starting on the very day you have your injection! This ensures that the blood does not stagnate in the leg veins, and also helps to open up accessory veins which will take over the drainage of blood from treated varicose ones.

You may find initially that walking causes you some pain or discomfort in the treated leg. Take some pain-killer (aspirin or paracetamol) and persist with your daily walking routine. You will find after a few days the discomfort will ease, and you will feel positively in better health from your daily exercise – both from your leg point of view and generally.

c *Clinic visits* Most doctors giving injection treatment to varicose veins will wish to see their patients again in one week following treatment. At this visit, as well as reviewing the continuing correct application of the compression bandage the success of the injection treatment can be assessed. Occasionally it may be necessary to give a further injection at this time to ensure that *all* the perforating veins have been treated. If all is well at this visit you will be asked to return at the end of six weeks. At this visit the bandages will be removed and you will be delighted to see your varicose veins are no more.

If at any time during the course of this six weeks you are concerned about anything to do with your leg, do not hesitate to contact the clinic – or your own doctor – for reassurance.

Possible complications

These are rare, and very many people have injection treatment to their varicose veins with absolutely no problem.

Pain A certain amount of pain around the injection site is to be expected during the first day or two. But pain-killers for a while and plenty of walking should be all that is necessary to ease this. Avoid standing still if at all possible – either walk or else sit with your bandaged leg raised.

Occasionally the compression bandages can become too tight and be uncomfortable. A visit to the clinic, or your doctor, for reapplication of the bandage, should relieve this problem. Whatever you do, *don't* remove the bandage altogether and leave it off. As mentioned before, the success of this form of treatment of varicose veins is very much dependent on the six weeks after-care – and adequate support bandage is a vital part of this.

Soreness over the site of the injection. This occasionally occurs due to the escape of a small amount of the irritant fluid into the surrounding tissues. If a small ulcer occurs, a dry dressing is all that is needed to heal this area.

Clotting in the deep veins of the leg is an extremely unusual occurrence after injection treatment. It can be completely avoided by adequate and continuing exercise during the whole of the six week period following the treatment.

Injection treatment is, in very many people, completely successful. But it does *not* ensure that you will never suffer from varicose veins again. The treated veins can dilate again (usually after many years) or different superficial veins can become varicosed. Under these circumstances the injection treatment can be repeated, or surgical treatment may need to be considered. In some people, a combination of both injection and surgical treatment will be considered the best way of dealing with their varicose veins.

Surgical treatment

The decision as to which treatment – injection or surgical – is the best for your particular case of varicose veins must obviously be left to the surgeon to whom your doctor has referred you. But in broad principle, surgical treatment is necessary for varicose veins which are a problem in the region of the thighs, as opposed to the lower part of the leg. Injection treatment in this area of the leg is less likely to be successful owing to the difficulty of applying a firm enough compression bandage.

Two further reasons why surgical treatment may be necessary is if:

1   Varicose veins are extensive and situated in both thigh and calf. Sometimes a 'mix' of both forms of treatment is thought preferable.

2   Injection treatment has proved unsuccessful in the past for some reason.

The following case history illustrates surgical treatment for varicose veins.

*   *   *

Dr Pilbeam sat down heavily in the surgeon's dressing-room.

'I shall have to get you to tie off my varicosities, Jim,' he said to his surgical colleague, who was pouring himself a welcome cup of coffee after a four-hour stint in the operating theatre.

'And who's going to give you the anaesthetic, Bill?' queried Jim Sharpe wryly, glancing down at his anaesthetist friend, who was rubbing an obviously aching leg. 'You can't do it yourself you know! – who are you going to trust?' he added with a twinkle in his eye. Bill Pilbeam, the senior anaesthetist at Blackmoor Hospital, had reached the top of his profession by sheer hard work and competence. His shrewd judgment was well respected throughout the group of hospitals. It would have to be an excellent anaesthetist indeed whom he would allow to give him an anaesthetic.

'Liz Goodman will do fine. I trained her myself.' Bill looked up, 'I'll come and see you in out-patients at the end of your clinic tomorrow – then you can decide what to do.'

At 5.30 p.m. the following day, the last sufferer at Jim Sharpe's Varicose Vein Clinic had departed. Sister Barrington was discussing a problem of an elderly patient with Mr Sharpe, when Dr Pilbeam appeared at the door.

Sister looked up in surprise. 'You're not a patient, I hope, Dr Pilbeam.'

'Indeed I am, Sister,' replied Bill Pilbeam. 'It's not always the ladies who need their varicose veins looked after, you know.'

'Sit down, Bill.' Jim Sharpe picked up his colleague's medical notes which were lying on a side table. 'Let's see – you had injections to your left calf seven years ago and a tie-off on your right leg three years ago. So which is bothering you now?'

Bill turned up his left trouser leg to show the knotted purple mass of varicose veins spreading from ankle to mid-calf.

'Speaks for itself, doesn't it?', he said wryly. 'And the skin's looking a bit delicate around here,' pointing at a patch of blotchy skin around his ankle joint.

Jim Sharpe examined the leg carefully, asking Bill to stand so that the damaged perforating veins could be accurately found. He straightened up after a few minutes. 'We'd better get these done as soon as possible Bill, or we'll be treating an ulcer sooner than you think. Why didn't you come to see me before?'

'Well, you know how it is – too much work, too little time, and one always hopes problems will go away!'

Bill Pilbeam's varicose veins were operated on as soon as space could be found in the tight theatre schedule. One week later he was back at work, anaesthetising once again for Jim Sharpe.

'Leg comfortable, Bill?' questioned Jim, as he slipped his hands into the surgical gloves held out by the theatre Sister.

'Fine, thanks – hopefully this will be the end of my varicose vein problems. I cannot think why I left it so long before consulting you. I should have known better!'

*   *   *

How surgical treatment works

There are two main forms of surgical treatment available, although the 'stripping' operation is less frequently used nowadays than the 'tie-off' operation.

1   The 'stripping' operation involves passing a fine wire up through the varicosed superficial vein, and actually pulling out the damaged portion of vein.

2   The 'tie-off' operation involves making a small incision over where the superficial varicosed vein pierces the fibrous sheath to join up with the deep venous system. The 'perforator' veins are then isolated, clamped and tied off with dissolvable stitches. Finally, the small skin wound is closed with sutures which will need removing at a later date. So you can see that the damaged veins are virtually removed from the system. There may be more than one situation on the thigh that requires this treatment.

How treatment will affect you

1   *At the time* Surgical treatment will require admission to hospital either:

a   for the day when the operation is done under a local anaesthetic,

b   for 2 or 3 days when the operation is done under a general anaesthetic.

The latter method, i.e. under a general anaesthetic, is the more usual way of performing this form of treatment.

You will be asked to arrive at the hospital ward on the morning of the day before your operation. While this may seem rather an unnecessary waste of time to you, there are a number of good reasons for this.

1   It allows the medical staff time to give you a thorough check over before you are given an anaesthetic. Usually a young newly-qualified doctor – the house-surgeon – will visit you to perform these checks. Your heart and lungs will be checked over, your blood-pressure will be taken, a sample of your urine will be checked and a sample of your blood will be

sent to the laboratory. In many hospitals, also, a chest X-ray will be done. These checks are important to ensure that you are fit before being given an anaesthetic. Every anaesthetic given has a tiny risk attached and the doctors (surgeons and anaesthetists) caring for you will need to be sure that you are fit.

2 The surgeon performing the operation will need to check on your varicose veins again before the operation. It may have been many weeks since he has seen you. (This task can be delegated to the surgeon's junior doctor, who will also be present at your operation and assisting with the procedure.)

3 Of vital importance also is the correct documentation to be added to your notes – your name, age, address etc. – all very necessary – ensuring that the correct operation is done. Very few mistakes are made in our hospitals, but without sufficient documentation, mistakes could occur. You will be issued with a plastic bracelet which has your name and age printed on it. This will be retained on your wrist throughout your stay in hospital.

4 Finally, the day's rest (however tedious it may seem to you as you take time out of a busy life) will enable you to get to know the staff of the ward on which you find yourself. It is good to be aware of a familiar face as you emerge from the deep sleep of your anaesthetic the following day.

The day of the operation

1 Nothing to eat or drink for at least twelve hours before you are due to have your anaesthetic. This means nothing at all by mouth from the last drink of the evening before if your operation is scheduled for the morning list. You will be allowed an early (very early!) cup of tea if your operation is due for the afternoon. This is important from the anaesthetic viewpoint. A full stomach can result in the inhalation to the lungs of possible vomit during the anaesthetic with potentially serious consequences. So under no circumstances be

tempted to sneak in either food or drink.

2   The hair on your legs and around the groin region will be shaved so that this does not get in the surgeon's way during the operation. Many hospitals allow patients to do this for themselves if they wish – disposable razors being provided. (The finished result will of course be checked by a member of the nursing staff!)

3   Then, finally, about an hour or so before your operation is due, your own night-clothes are removed and you are given a white operating gown to put on. An injection will then be given. This will make you feel pleasurably drowsy, or may even send you off to sleep altogether. So you may, or may not, be aware of being transferred to a trolley and wheeled to the operating theatre.

4   In the anaesthetic room next door to the operating theatre, the anaesthetist (a doctor specially trained in this branch of medicine) will be waiting to give your anaesthetic. A tiny prick in your arm is all you will remember until you wake up again in an hour or two, the operation completed and your leg bandaged with only some discomfort to feel – rather as if you had given yourself a hefty blow on the leg! It is then back to the ward for you, where a further pain-killing injection will be given if the discomfort becomes severe. You will then probably drift off to sleep again for several hours, to wake again feeling more your usual self.

The succeeding week or two

a   You will be allowed home within a couple of days of your operation, depending on how quickly you recover from the anaesthetic. Many surgeons are happy to let their patients return home the day following the operation.

b   The bandages on your leg should be left in place until the time comes to remove the stitches. This is usually after five to six days. These stitches can be removed either at hospital or in your doctor's surgery by his practice nurse.

c Again – as following injection treatment – walking is of vital importance in ensuring the best possible success of the operation. So set off on your daily walk as soon as you possibly can after your return home. Try to build up to the magic three miles a day within the next week or so. And, again when you are sitting be sure to prop your legs up on a chair or some other convenient piece of furniture.

d Depending on your work you may well be able to return to your job after a week. This will depend very much, of course, on the nature of your work. Office employment could be continued as long as you can sit with your leg rested in a comfortable horizontal position as you work. (Remember, too, to take time out to fit in your daily walk.) More active strenuous jobs will probably need two or three weeks off work to ensure that the wound, or wounds, in your leg is fully healed. Men who drive – perhaps heavy vehicles – for a living will also need to be sure that they are able to move their legs with sufficient alacrity to respond to any emergency situation. For such workers two or three weeks off work may also be necessary.

These then are the various treatments available to deal with varicose veins. Each case must be looked at individually and the best treatment decided upon. But hopefully whatever is done there will be much improvement both in appearance and comfort.

The next chapter will discuss the complications that can occur with untreated varicose veins and what can be done to help if these complications do occur.

5

Possible complications of Varicose Veins

Talk to people about varicose veins and you will realize that it is the complications about which they are most worried. Nearly everyone knows at least one old lady who suffers much pain and discomfort from varicose ulcers that will not heal. Thrombosis in a vein with resulting painful inflammation is also a risk that many people automatically assume is inevitable with varicose veins. And how many first aid books – and examiners – talk about serious haemorrhage from a varicose vein?

While, of course, all these events can happen, it is by no means a certainty that your particular clutch of varicose veins will proceed to have any of these problems. In fact for every 100 cases of uncomplicated varicose veins on which your doctor advises, he will only see one or two people with any one of the four possible complications. Most people who attend their doctor will be asking for help with either the appearance of their varicose veins or for relief from aching, and perhaps swollen legs. The swelling which sometimes arises around the ankles of people with varicose veins is due to the back pressure into the capillaries and hence leakage of fluid into the tissues of the lower leg. This is also a potent factor in the heavy ache in the legs at the end of a long day on one's feet. This swelling will soon disperse if you raise your legs into the horizontal position. Such a swelling could perhaps also be classified as a 'complication' of varicose veins. But fortunately it is easily cured by 'taking the weight off your feet' – quite literally!

But now a look at the more severe possible complications of varicose veins in turn, how they are caused, and what treatment needs to be instituted to clear up, or alleviate, the problem.

Pigmentation

Pigmentation is the alteration in the colour of the skin. The pigmentation due to varicose veins is invariably seen in the lower part of the leg, below an obvious cluster of varicose veins. As well as being termed 'varicose pigmentation', this discoloration can be known as 'varicose eczema' or 'varicose dermatitis'. Strictly speaking both these latter names are incorrect. 'Eczema' implies an allergy factor and 'dermatitis' means an inflammation of the skin. Neither of these processes play a part in the pigmentation seen as a result of varicose veins.

How pigmentation is caused

Again, it is the villain of the piece at work again – that high back pressure down from the veins into the tiny capillaries, those 'link-men' between the arterial and venous part of the circulatory system. When this pressure becomes excessive some of the red blood corpuscles are forced out through the thin walls of the capillaries into the tissue of the leg. The red pigment in the corpuscles, containing iron, then breaks down further and is deposited in the tissues immediately beneath the surface of the skin. It is this substance which gives the typical purplish discoloration.

Treatment for varicose pigmentation

Regretfully, once the skin has become heavily discoloured there is little that can be done to improve the situation. The pigment from the red blood corpuscles is well and truly settled in the skin cells and those of the underlying tissues. When this stage is reached, covering cosmetic creams are the best way of camouflaging these – sometimes unsightly – stains.

But if you have sought help for your varicose veins early enough it is unlikely that this pigmentation will even occur. And even if a small amount of discoloration can be seen, early and adequate treatment of the offending varicose veins can improve the condition – and certainly will prevent it worsening.

So once again, the message is prevention. In spite of the fact that some factors in the incidence of varicose veins cannot be altered – sex and family for example – remember that there is still much that you can do both to reduce symptoms and to prevent complications of varicose veins (for further discussion on this, see Chapter 6).

Ulceration

Varicose ulcers do not arise overnight. These unpleasant, sore lesions are the result of long-standing varicose veins. With adequate treatment of varicose veins and scrupulous care of legs prone to varicose vein complications, most people can avoid ulcers. It is older people, who have difficulty (for many different reasons) in moving around who can be at greater risk of developing a varicose ulcer. So extra care of legs amongst senior citizens must be an important item in their daily routine of physical care.

Why ulceration occurs

The basic reason causing the skin surface in a leg below a varicose vein to break down is poor nutrition of the skin and underlying tissue. The stagnant blood, with its high back pressure in a bunch of varicose veins presses on and contorts the arteries supplying the skin in this region. Because of this diminished supply of arterial blood the tissues are denied their full quota of oxygen and nutrients for healthy living and repair. The skin becomes thin and brittle and patches of pigmentation may appear. Unhealthy skin due to this reason becomes itchy. And it only needs a brisk scratch of the skin to control the irritation to rub off the top layer of skin. (A minor bang against the leg of a chair, for example, can have exactly the same effect.) Normal healthy skin can easily cope with such minor injuries by healing quickly and painlessly. But the poorly oxygenated and comparatively starved skin below a severe, untreated varicose vein does not heal so rapidly. All too quickly this trivial scratch or break in the skin becomes an ulcer. And unless immediate and adequate treatment is given, this ulcer can increase in size and persist for many months, causing much pain and discomfort.

(In elderly people – in whom ulcers are most likely to occur – the doctor must make certain that it really is varicose veins that are the cause of the ulceration. Lower leg ulceration can also be caused by a poor arterial blood supply. The tiny arteries to the lower limbs can become thickened and partially blocked. This has the effect of – again – poor nutrition of the skin of this part of the leg. So ulceration can result, but for a different basic reason. Both conditions – varicose veins and arterial disease – can exist together. So it is important to sort out in each individual just what is causing the problem. Briefly, with arterial disease, the foot will be permanently cold and the pulses (felt behind the knee and at the ankle) will be weaker than usual. But that is another – fascinating – story . . .)

Treatment for a varicose ulcer

The rationale behind the treatment of a varicose ulcer is to improve the blood supply to the ulcerated part. Then, the body's own mechanisms should be able to heal the ulcer. To do this the back pressure from the varicose veins on to the adjacent arterial blood supply must be relieved. And this brings us back again to our four-pronged method – as in the generalised treatment for varicose veins.

1   *Raising the leg* above the level of the heart so that the veins will be emptied by gravity is the most obvious way of relieving the back pressure. Fine at night – remember to prop your leg up on a couple of pillows if you do not fancy raising the end of your bed. But none of us are able to stay in this position all the time. (And, indeed, it would do the rest of our bodies little good if we did.) So some other method must be used to force the stagnant blood in the varicose veins onward on its journey back to the heart.

2   *Firm bandaging* And I mean really *firm* bandaging, with either a special elasticised bandage or with firm Elastoplast. Support stockings, crêpe bandages or Tubigrip bandage are just not strong enough to give firm enough control.

You will need to attend your doctor's surgery to have your leg bandaged properly. Quite apart from the difficulty of bandaging your own leg, it needs a fair degree of expertise to apply a firm elastic covering. The bandage must be put on firmly and tightly – but not so tight as to jeopardise the arterial blood supply to the lower leg – the very thing you are trying to improve. The pressure exerted over all the leg must be consistent as well. A bandage which has a slack section in the middle is of little use – the very thing that is likely to cause further stagnation of blood in a damaged vein.

Once applied (and this must be done with the leg raised so that the veins are as empty as possible) the bandage must remain in position until the healing of the ulcer is complete. Obviously, the bandage will need to be removed at regular intervals to chart the progress of the ulcer, and to ensure that the pressure remains firm and consistent.

(A word of warning about the use of Elastoplast bandages. If you are one of those unfortunate people who are allergic to 'sticky plasters' do let your doctor know before he orders an

Elastoplast bandage to be applied to your leg. The last thing you want is an allergic rash on top of your varicose ulcer! Under these circumstances, either an elasticated bandage will be used, or your leg will be encased in either an ordinary gauze bandage or a special non-allergic bandage before being covered by the Elastoplast bandaging.)

3 *Regular walking* Don't think you have got out of taking a daily three mile or so walk just because you have a varicose ulcer! The firm bandaging will do much to prevent blood stagnating in your varicose veins. But the beneficial effect of the regular 'muscle-pump' on the deep veins of the leg – and so also on the superficial varicose veins – must never be under-estimated. So – if you are able – walk as much as you can every day. (And when not walking, sit with your leg raised to a horizontal position.)

4 *Watch your weight* And that means losing some if you are overweight! Pads of fat around the pelvis and thighs all exert extra pressure on the blood supply to your lower legs. And this means stagnant blood in varicosed veins and diminished arterial blood supply and poorly nourished skin. So, although weight-watching should be part of your preventative measures, in the event of a varicose ulcer developing, this assumes added importance (see Chapter 6 for further discussion on this aspect of the varicose vein story).

These then are the immediate forms of treatment necessary to control – and cure – a varicose ulcer. Once this has been done, attention must be paid to the root cause of the problem – the varicose veins causing the poor nutrition of the skin. These must then be dealt with either by injection or surgical treatment. You must always be on your guard against further situations that could result in another varicose ulcer. Support stockings, weight-control as well as keeping up the good habit of active exercise daily must all be part of your life-style in the future.

Phlebitis (or thrombo-phlebitis)

Most people have heard of 'phlebitis'. It conjures up a picture of an elderly lady sitting with a heavily bandaged leg propped up on a stool for months on end! There is some degree of truth in this mental vision, but men can also suffer from an attack of phlebitis and the condition resolves itself in weeks rather than months.

What is phlebitis?

Phlebitis occurs in a vein when a clot (or thrombus) blocks off the vessel. This sets up an inflammatory process in the tissues surrounding the vein. ('Itis' at the end of any word means that an inflammatory process is occurring.) There are two types of inflammatory processes commonly occurring in the body. One type involves bacteria or viruses. The inflammatory process under these conditions is the body's reaction to these invaders, and is an important part of the body's defence mechanisms. Antibiotics can help in the destruction of invading bacteria (they have *no* action against viruses) and so can be extremely helpful in inflammatory conditions due to bacteria. The second type of inflammation is a chemical reaction to some unusual circumstances in the body – in the case of phlebitis, the clot in the varicosed vein.

A similar situation arises when you bang some part of your body against a hard object without breaking the skin. This sets up an inflammatory process in which no invading organisms are present.

But to get back to phlebitis. You will be only too aware that something unusual is going on in association with your varicosed vein if you have phlebitis. The area around the clotted (or thrombosed) vein will be red and painful and exquisitely tender to touch. This area will correspond exactly to the course of the involved vein.

Treatment for phlebitis

This is simple but time-consuming! You must rest your leg – either in bed or sitting with it propped horizontally on a chair – until the inflammation has settled. This may take three or four weeks. You will probably need a supply of pain-killing tablets (aspirin or paracetamol) initially to control the pain. Also a light crêpe bandage (put on starting from the base of the toes up to the knee) may make your leg feel more comfortable.

When the most severe part of the inflammation has settled, you should start walking short distances. But remember not to stand for any length of time or sit with your leg down. Either walk or sit or lie with your leg up must be your rule until the condition has subsided.

No one knows exactly what makes the blood clot in a particular varicose vein. The best way of prevention is support stockings and dedicated daily walking if you suffer from varicose veins of any severity.

To many people a clot in a leg vein can be a worrying phenomenon. Most people have heard stories of the clot 'breaking away' and travelling to other vital areas of the body. This happens *very* rarely with a thrombo-phlebitis in a superficial varicose vein. It is when a blood clot occurs in one of the deep veins that there is a greater possibility of this occurring. Clotting in these deep veins can happen after surgical operations or after a major accident involving the legs. But as the inflammation settles, the blood clot will gradually be absorbed giving no further problems. In fact the varicose vein in the area may have improved in appearance due to the blood flow stopping in this particular vein.

Haemorrhage

Haemorrhage from varicose veins is a favourite example of venous haemorrhage in first-aid books. And a very good example it is when discussing the control of haemorrhage. But to those people who suffer from severe varicose veins, this can imply that haemorrhage from varicose veins is a common event. And this can be worrying. The truth is that haemorrhage from varicose veins is a comparatively *rare* event.

How haemorrhage can occur

Haemorrhage only occurs when a varicose vein receives a severe direct blow or the skin over the vein is snagged on some sharp object. As we have seen, the skin overlying severe varicose veins tends to be thin and brittle due to poor nourishment. So when some injury, perhaps relatively trivial, occurs at this particular point the skin breaks easily. The dilated thin-walled veins, being near the surface of the skin can also be involved in the injury. The blood, being stagnate in this region and also under considerable back pressure due to the failed valves (and also the upright position), hence pours out frighteningly.

Treatment of haemorrhage from an injured varicose vein

1 Raise the affected leg until it is higher than the level of the heart. Almost miraculously, it will seem, the flow of blood from the wound will diminish. Merely counteracting the effect of gravity, and thus relieving the high back pressure on the vein will have a dramatic effect.

2 Take the nearst available clean object (handkerchief, tea-towel if no 'made-to-measure' dressing in a first-aid box is to hand) and hold this firmly over the bleeding vein. Exert firm pressure with your hand. Keep the dressing in place with a bandage of some kind – adding extra dressings over the top of the original one if the bleeding should still be persistent.

3 Call an ambulance or get someone to take you to the accident-and-emergency department of your nearest hospital. But remember to keep the injured leg high above

the level of your heart and to maintain the firm pressure.

At the hospital treatment will very much depend on the size of the wound and the state of the surrounding skin. Stitches are very often an unsuitable form of treatment due to the latter, so other forms of conservative treatment have to be considered. But be prepared to sit with your leg up for several days, giving your bodily mechanisms a chance to heal the wound that has been sustained in a less-than-perfect tissue. Great care must be taken to ensure that the wound is completely healed before full activities are undertaken again. Inadequate healing can result in the formation of a persistent ulcer, which can be difficult to treat satisfactorily. Remember that patience for a few extra days following this type of injury can save more long-standing problems.

The following case histories illustrate what happens when injuries are sustained.

*   *   *

'That leg looks painful, Mrs Brooks.' Mrs Conway, long-term proprietress of one of the last-remaining village stores, looked anxiously as her customer lowered her not inconsiderable bulk into the chair beside the counter. 'Whatever have you done to it?' she continued, bending down to investigate the reddened, swollen swelling on Mrs Brooks' shin.

'I fell up the steps in the garden, Mrs Conway,' confessed Mrs Brooks. 'Stupid thing to do! I must admit it was painful at the time. It seemed to be healing well until yesterday. But now it looks as if there is something in it – doesn't it?'

'You had better make an appointment to see Dr Harris – soon!' Mrs Conway remarked, getting to her feet. 'We don't want you in a wheelchair!'

The following day Mrs Brooks limped into Dr Harris's consulting room.

'Sit down, Mrs Brooks. I don't see you very often. What's the trouble?'

'Well, doctor – the garden step attacked my shin a week ago! It was healing well. But now it is red and swollen – and painful. I am wondering if there is something in it?' Mrs Brookes grunted with the effort of removing her stocking.

'Let me help,' said Dr Harris, 'all that extra weight you are carrying is not helping, you know.' He bent to loosen the cotton bandage that Mrs Brookes had tied loosely round her leg.

'Oh, yes. I see what you mean. It certainly is not healing properly. No, there is nothing in it – it looks quite clean.' Dr Harris gently swabbed around the red, swollen area on Mrs Brookes's leg. 'You have an ulcer developing here, due to the bang on your shin. There is a poor blood supply around that area of your leg. And with those varicose veins that you have lower down on your leg,' Dr Harris pointed to the mass of purple swellings on Mrs Brookes's calf, '– the poor old skin is not getting too much blood to it so that healing can occur. So –' Dr Harris stood up, hands on hips, '– three things you must do, Mrs Brookes. First of all, let's get that skin healed. Firm bandaging for at least six weeks – not a day less! And sit with that leg up when you are not walking about. My nurse will bandage it for you. Then after it is healed, we must do something about your varicose veins. But meanwhile –' and Dr Harris's tone became firm, '– you must try and lose some of that weight. I would guess that you are somewhere around fifteen stone?'

'Well – yes! – fifteen and a half, actually!' Mrs Brookes confessed. 'I've been meaning to get some of it off for ages. But this will make me try harder.'

Half-an-hour later, her leg firmly bandaged, Mrs Brookes called in at Mrs Conway's shop.

'What's the verdict then, Mrs Brookes?' called Mrs Conway from the top of a step-ladder where she was restocking her shelves.

'An ulcer developing due to the bang on my shin and the poor blood supply, partly due to my varicose veins. So – it is to be bandaged tightly for six weeks – I'm to go back to the health centre and have it re-done when it gets loose. Then Dr Harris is going to do something about my varicose veins. And I've got to lose some weight!' Mrs Brookes added quietly.

'I heard that!' Mrs Conway came down from the ladder. 'So put those biscuits down. I'll weigh you up a pound of these delicious Cox's apples instead.'

Six weeks later Mrs Brookes's leg was fully healed. She confidently stepped on to the scales in Dr Harris's consulting room.

'A stone off already, Doctor,' she said, proudly. 'And I certainly feel much better for it.'

'Well done, Mrs Brookes! Keep up the good work. I've put your name down on the waiting list at the hospital varicose vein clinic to have those veins injected.'

*   *   *

'Come quickly Mum! Gran's fallen over by the apple tree – and her leg's bleeding like billy-ho!'

The white, anxious face of nine-year-old Jonathan Lowth appeared over the kitchen window-sill where Jenny Lowth was busy peeling potatoes. Dropping the knife, Jenny picked up a clean tea-towel and shaking the surplus water off her hands, ran out of the back door.

Under the apple tree she found her seventy-year-old mother sitting on the edge of an upturned chair clutching at the calf of her left leg. Blood was oozing between her fingers in a steady flow, darkening the grass in an ever-widening circle.

'I – I – think I've caught my varicose vein, Jenny. The chair tipped up and dug into my leg. It – it – does seem to be

62

bleeding rather a lot, dear. . . .' Mrs Beckett's voice quavered into silence.

Jenny's mind clicked back to the first aid lecture on bleeding she had attended the year before when her firm had asked for volunteers for a first aid course.

'Lie down, mother – on your back – Jon – move that chair and prop Gran's foot on it.' She was folding the tea-towel into a neat, thick pad as she helped her mother down on to the grass. 'All right now? – goodness you are heavy!' She gasped, as the full weight of her mother's not inconsiderable shoulders descended into her arms.

'Right now – leg up as high as you can.' And Jenny placed her make-shift dressing firmly over the wound in her mother's leg.

'Coo – it's like magic, Mum!' Jon stood wide-eyed. 'It's hardly bleeding at all now!'

'That's partly because Gran's leg is up in the air, Jon,' Jenny explained. 'Can you hold this pad on tightly while I go and phone for an ambulance. There's a good lad.'

And Jenny ran back to the house to dial 999.

Two hours later, leg neatly bandaged and propped up in a chair in the sitting-room, Mrs Beckett was sipping a welcome cup of tea.

'I'm very glad you did that first aid course, Jenny. It certainly came in useful this afternoon.'

'I would have been very worried if I hadn't known what to do,' admitted Jenny. 'But now we will have to work out your diet, mother!' She added briskly. 'The doctor at the hospital was right when he said all that weight is no good for you or your varicose veins!'

'That's exactly what Dr Cummings said when I saw her a few weeks ago about treatment for the veins,' Mrs Beckett sighed. 'She said she wouldn't think of sending me for treatment until I lost some weight. So – when should I start?' she added in a questioning voice.

'Now!' said Jenny as she gently took the biscuit that was half-way to her mother's mouth out of her hand.

Six months later, and three stone lighter, Mrs Beckett walked the mile to her daughter's house.

'I do feel fitter, you know Jenny,' she said. 'Without all that weight! And the doctor at the hospital said he would start treatment on my varicose veins next week. So perhaps our rather worrying afternoon last summer was not all bad luck after all!'

*   *   *

These, then, are the complications that can occur from varicose veins. But it must be stressed again that these conditions are by no means common events occurring in all people who suffer from varicose veins. And they never appear suddenly – apart from haemorrhage, of course. Varicose veins will have been present for many years, and hopefully adequate treatment will have been given early enough to prevent complications occurring.

The next chapter will discuss various ways in which you can reduce the effects of varicose veins on your own particular life-style. With a few minor changes in your daily routine, you may well not only reduce the discomfort in your varicose veins, but could improve your general health as well!

6

Self Help for Varicose Vein Sufferers

While it is impossible to ensure that one specific individual never suffers from varicose veins, much can be done to reduce the discomfort due to varicose veins. Also, preventative measures can very much help in ensuring that minimal varicose veins remain minimal. As a spin-off, the life-style that helps varicose veins is also one that does much for your general health.

As we have seen in early chapters, whether or not any particular individual will suffer from varicose veins – perhaps even as early as in their late teenage years – depends very much on their family history and their sex. And it is impossible to alter either of these two factors! But there are three main areas which, with a little perseverance, will do much to reducing any varicose vein problems to a minimum.

Exercise

General exercise

We have seen how important a part walking plays in the care of the legs following either injection or surgical treatment. As well as the massaging action of the muscles during the actual walking process, the 'tone' of the muscles is permanently improved by regular walking. This in turn will improve the support given to the blood vessels of the leg when it is necessary to stand still. The ideal three miles a day – as necessary after surgery or injection of varicose veins – may not be possible to fit into a busy day's schedule. But an effort to walk a mile or two every day will do much to benefit your legs – and your general health as well.

Other forms of general activity involving leg muscles – from cycling to swimming and playing active games such as badminton or table tennis – will have the same beneficial effect. So why not look round locally and find out what is available in your local neighbourhood? Who knows – you may find yourself involved in a whole new range of interesting hobbies and activities.

Specific leg exercises

While it is not always possible to take a two-mile walk just when you feel inclined, it is often possible to do one or two exercises specifically geared to improve the circulation in your legs. The exercises designed for the lower part of the leg (the commonest situation for most people's varicose veins) can be incorporated into a busy day's schedule. The ones which exercise the upper part of the leg will need the privacy of your home. But well worth sparing ten minutes or so to do every day.

Exercises for calf muscles

1 *Walk on tiptoe* whenever possible! It sounds simple – and indeed is simple – but this is very effective in tightening up those calf muscles, and so massaging the blood up in the veins more efficiently.

(As an added bonus, this way of moving will stretch and strengthen the small muscles of the feet. This in turn will ensure that feet have a good arch and do not become flat!)
2 As you sit – either at work or at home in the evening – *circle your foot* round and round several times in each direction. Take big, wide sweeps in all directions. As you do this, put a hand on your calf muscles and note how they alternately tighten and relax as your foot moves. Do not just confine this exercise to the leg that has the varicose veins. Both ankles and legs will benefit from the extra muscle

strength and joint mobility this will give if done regularly.

Exercise for thigh muscles

1   Sit with your legs out in front of you, with about six inches between your ankles. Starting with your right leg, lift this off the ground as far as you can with comfort; hold this position whilst you count up to five and then relax. Repeat with the other leg and then repeat the sequence again with both legs five times. Remember not to lean back on your hands as you do this exercise.

2   Lie on your back, arms by your sides; raise your legs and with each leg, make bicycling movements in the air. Circle your legs about ten times, if you can manage this without discomfort.

(Neither of these exercises should be performed if you have any heart, lung or joint condition which makes active movement inadvisable. If in any doubt, check with your doctor before attempting the exercises.)

There are other, equally suitable, leg exercises that can be done. You may like to try a few different ones suggested in magazines or books, or possibly ones advised by the physiotherapy department at your local hospital. But remember that to reap the full benefit, any exercise must be done on a regular basis. It is no use at all rushing out to walk three miles and then doing your leg exercises and collapsing into a chair thinking that is adequate exercise for this week! Much better to walk one mile each day and practise one exercise each day. After a week or two this will become part of your daily routine – and how much better for it you will feel. Muscles all over your body are strengthened, heart and lungs work to greater efficiency following a daily walk and circulation is improved in the vast network of all your blood vessels, including those damaged ones in your varicose veins.

While still on the exercise theme, do not forget that standing still for long periods of time is the very worst thing for your varicose veins. Some people's work may necessitate them standing for long hours. If this is so for you, and your varicose veins are causing you much discomfort, move from foot to foot at regular intervals during the day. Make every excuse to walk a few yards, or consciously to stretch up on tiptoe every now and again. Remember, too, to wear support stockings. All these manoeuvres will ensure that the blood is kept moving in the veins of your leg.

Also do not forget to raise your leg to the horizontal position when you are able to sit down. Finding a convenient stool or chair should be your aim when you are able to have a break from standing. Sitting with your legs crossed is also 'out' if your varicose veins are severe. The blood cannot be expected to flow smoothly upwards if veins are flattened and kinked.

Lose some weight!

It is thought that at least half the adult population of Britain is overweight to some degree. Exercise, if kept up regularly will go some way to keeping weight gain under control. But the basic cause of overweight is eating too much for the needs of your body. The amount of food needed to keep one particular human body in good health is very individual. Every person has a different 'metabolic rate'. This is basically a measure of how effectively 'fuel' (in the way of food) is used in our bodies. We all know of people who eat everything and anything they want, and do not put on a pound. And we all know of people who if they ate exactly the same diet day by day would be of an enormous size within a month or two! (And these differences can sometimes be seen even in two members of the same family.) Heredity does of course play a part here as in every other physical characteristic. So if you come from a family who puts weight on easily, chances are high that you too will have to watch your weight as the years go by. Remember, too, that family eating patterns are also passed on from generation to generation. If the family has enjoyed big, weight-inducing meals for years, a deliberate effort will have to be made to alter the tradition if you are anxious to avoid overweight.

Losing weight is all very fine in theory, but far more difficult to put into practice. Ample evidence is given of this by the multitude of articles, leaflets, magazines and not to mention whole books on the subject of how to lose weight. Everyone has there own favourite slimming diet – which may or may not work! It is very important, however, to avoid 'crash' slimming courses. Whilst these may indeed be successful in causing the weight to drop off, your health can suffer as a result. Too rapid slimming can:

1   alter the body's chemistry; leaving the way open for infections to take hold;
2   anaemia, too, can result if adequate amounts of suitable food are not taken on a regular basis,
3   and one of the more worrying aspects of slimming is the ease with which a slimmer can slip into the condition known as 'anorexia nervosa'. This is a condition (most often seen in adolescent girls and young women, but older people are by no means excluded) in which food is avoided almost completely. The girl still sees her body as gross and fat, even though she is painfully thin and continues to insist she needs to be slimmer. All kinds of ruses to avoid food – by hiding it and inducing vomiting after eating for example – are thought up. Closely associated with anorexia nervosa is a condition known as 'bulimia'. The sufferer will have bouts of eating enormous amounts of food alternating with self-induced vomiting. These 'binges' are alternated with weeks when food is refused altogether. Both these conditions can have

potentially serious consequences and will need skilled medical treatment to correct the upset in the biochemistry of the body.

These are extreme conditions associated with slimming of course, but nevertheless ones to be remembered and avoided. Slimming treatments need to be done in moderation, with due regard to a balanced diet.

How our diet is made up

There are five basic groups of food required by our bodies every day for complete health.

1 *Carbohydrates* These are the sweet, sugary foods that put on weight as soon as you look at them – sticky pastries, puddings, biscuits, sweets of all kinds, fruit squashes and 'pop' to mention just a few. By cutting out most of these items from your diet you will be doing much to lose weight. (You will also, incidentally, be doing much to promote positive health in many organs of your body.)

2 *Protein* A certain amount of protein is necessary every day adequately to cope with the repair of our bodily cells. Protein foods are meat, eggs, fish and cheese. These foods contain all the amino-acids (the building blocks of cells) necessary for this maintenance schedule. These are known as first-class proteins. Second-class proteins are to be found in peas, beans, lentils etc. Comparatively large amounts of these latter protein foods have to be eaten to ensure an adequate protein intake.

3 *Fats* This constituent of our diet can be taken in the form of animal or vegetable fat. A typical Western diet often contains too much fat, particularly if cream, ice-cream, lashings of butter and unskimmed milk are all part of the daily eating routine.

4   *Vitamins and minerals* Both these groups of substances are necessary for health, *but* only in small daily amounts. If an adequate diet in other respects is being eaten daily, there is no need for vitamin or mineral supplements.

5   *Roughage and water* Not exactly a group of foods as in the other necessary components of a daily diet, but nevertheless important in terms of a weight-reducing diet. Roughage in the form of wholemeal bread and cereals and fibrous fruit and vegetables not only keeps the bowels in a healthy condition, but also fills up those hungry, empty spaces that can make dieting so difficult. Water, too, is a vital component of everyday living and the minimum required by every adult daily is two pints. Drinking extra water will also have the effect of reducing hunger pangs! But do not take this to extremes and live on a water-only diet. 'Moderation' in everything is the key word to successful dieting. (Also be sure that your 'drink' does not consist of squashes or fizzy drinks with a high carbohydrate intake. This will defeat the whole object of drinking a little extra fluid.)

Broad guidelines on a weight reducing diet

Bearing in mind the necessity of including some foods from each of the five groups, the way to lose weight is to eat less – and that means less of everything! In this way, there will be no chance that your diet will become unbalanced. An unbalanced diet means that your body will be lacking in some necessary component. Obviously, if your diet has been heavily biased towards lots of cream cakes and buttery crumpets, for example, you should cut down markedly on this group. (In fact, omit these foods altogether, except for one day every week or so when you allow yourself a 'treat'. You will be surprised, though, at how quickly you will cease to enjoy these types of foods.) Similarly, if you have been living on chocolate bars, bread-and-butter and sticky buns, this emphasis on the carbohydrate grouping must also be adjusted.

With a little knowledge of the constituents of different foods, eating sensibly (and this will mean losing weight) is really a matter of common-sense – and will-power!

The '*Traffic-light diet*' is always one that has appealed to me – in reality for children! But adults can learn much from the rules.

The '*red*' foods are the ones that spell 'danger' for overweight people. This group must include sweets, biscuits, cream, ice-cream, sugar, cakes and other similar foods.

The '*amber*' foods are those that can be eaten with caution – necessary in small quantities daily for health, but not to be over-indulged in. This means milk and dishes made with quantities of milk, cheese and cream, root vegetables of all kinds – potatoes, carrots, parsnips etc. – should be eaten sparingly. Beware, also, those tempting sauces that make an evening meal out such a treat, and save these for very special occasions only.

The '*green*' foods are those that can be eaten freely. Green vegetables, fruit, particularly apples and citrus fruit, white meat and eggs.

Again, of course, common sense must prevail. It is not sensible to live solely on eggs and cabbage for example (and very unappetising too!). But a varied selection of foods daily with less emphasis on the 'red' and 'amber' foods will do much to shed a few pounds steadily every month.

An example of a suitable daily diet would be:

Breakfast   Half a grapefruit or fruit juice, boiled egg if wished, two slices wholemeal bread with a scraping of butter or margarine, tea or coffee with a minimum of skimmed milk.

Mid-morning   Black coffee, tea with lemon, 'low-calorie' drink or meat extract drink.

Lunch	Cottage cheese/lean meat with salad, fresh fruit.
Tea	Tea with lemon (or minimum milk).
Supper	Clear soup or fruit juice, fish/lean meat with two small potatoes and green vegetables, fresh fruit salad or 1 oz cheese with dry biscuit, black coffee or minimum of skimmed milk.

Obviously you should vary this throughout the week, by substituting other foods from the appropriate groups. But use this as a basic guide-line.

You will be doing well if you lose 2–4 lbs during the first week of your slimming diet. Every week after this, aim at losing 1–2 lbs regularly until you reach your target weight. (The initial greater loss is due to the loss of excess water held in the tissues.)

A further way of helping to reduce weight is to remember the 'triple' three-pronged attack on 'cooking', 'meals' and 'type of food' (or CMT).

Cooking

1 Boil, bake, grill or steam as many foods as you can. Cut out fried foods altogether and keep roasts to a minimum.
2 If you do roast, never add any further fat to the cooking. For example, let a joint of meat roast – in foil or an enclosed tin – in its own fat and juices.
3 Use yoghurt instead of cream or excess oil in dressings.

Meals

1 Eat three meals a day on a regular basis.
2 Do not be tempted to miss meals. This will only result in you being extra hungry later, and also could well damage your health if continued for too long.
3 Eat nothing in between meals – no added biscuit or bun with mid-morning drink for example.

Type of food

1 Cut down on the 'stop' group of foods.
2 Try to eat at least three pieces of fruit every day. (Your half grapefruit for breakfast could count as one piece, for example.)
3 Fibre foods up – and fat foods down – is a good rule to remember. Not only your weight will benefit, but also bowel and blood-vessels, by this rule.

The only other ingredient to be added to your plan is 'will-power'!

Care after any episodes of complications due to varicose veins

As has been seen in previous chapters, it is by no means inevitable that complications will occur if you have varicose veins. In fact the whole aim of self-help and treatment is to reduce to a minimum the possibility of this situation. But there will probably always be those few unfortunate people who will suffer one or other of the four main complications of varicose veins – pigmentation, ulceration, thrombo-phlebitis or haemorrhage. And it is especially important to take extra care of your legs following any such episode.

1 Conscientious wearing of adequate *support stockings* after ulceration will do much to prevent the tissues breaking down again. Remember to put on your stocking *before* you get out of bed. And remember also to check regularly that elasticity of your support stockings. Regular – and necessary – washing will gradually weaken the fabric. Support stockings will need to be renewed every three months or so if they are worn regularly on a daily basis.
2 Practise until it becomes an ingrained habit of *sitting with your legs up*. Not always possible, I know, in social situations, but certainly at home do keep an extra chair or

stool handy on which to prop your legs. If your work involves sitting all day it is well worth investigating possibilities of finding *something* on which to support your leg that has had problems.

Also remember not to cross your legs, at knee or ankle, when you do have to sit in a chair for any length of time.

3   *Walking* to tone up those leg muscles to fulfil their task of 'pumping' the blood satisfactorily through the veins. After the initial period of rest necessary to heal an ulcer or to settle down an episode of thrombo-phlebitis, a daily walk will do much to reduce the possibility of a recurrence to a minimum. Start yourself off gently at first, gradually building up your distance until you are – ideally – walking around two or three miles every day.

All these aspects of care following complication are also relevant, of course, to care of yourself following operative or injection treatment of your varicose veins – as has been seen in previous chapters.

4   Finally – and this applies whether or not you have had any complications to your varicose veins – do take care that the leg that has the varicose veins *stays out of the way of injury*, as far as is possible. Fortunately, one of the commonest places for varicose veins to occur, on the inside of the calves of the legs, is largely protected from injury. But nevertheless take care that sharp edges to furniture do not damage this particularly vulnerable part of your body. Remember an injury to this part of your leg can be one of the factors in producing an ulcer, which in turn can be difficult to heal.

Varicose veins are not a life-threatening condition. But nevertheless their presence can cause much discomfort throughout many years. If you add to this the pain and inconvenience that can be caused by any one of the complications that can occur, it is well worth doing all you can to avoid the latter and reduce discomfort to a minimum. Your doctor and surgeon can do much to relieve your problems. But after their work has been done, the ball is firmly back in your court.

Index